# Plant-Based Nutrition for Beginners

## The Essential Guide to Achieving Optimal Health naturally with constant vegetable consumption

Graham Julian Oliver

**Published by Graham Julian Oliver**

# Disclaimer

This book, *Plant-Based Nutrition for Beginners: The Essential Guide to Achieving Optimal Health Naturally with Constant Vegetable Consumption*, is intended solely for informational and educational purposes. It is not intended to provide medical, health, or nutritional advice, nor should it replace consultation with qualified healthcare professionals. Readers are encouraged to consult their physician or other healthcare providers before making any significant changes to their diet, exercise regimen, or lifestyle, especially if they have any pre-existing health conditions.

While every effort has been made to ensure the accuracy and reliability of the information within this book, the author and publisher make no representations or warranties, express or implied, regarding the content's completeness, accuracy, or suitability for any purpose. The author and publisher disclaim any liability or responsibility for any adverse effects, losses, or damages arising directly or indirectly from the use or application of the contents of this book.

Furthermore, this book contains references to certain products, websites, organizations, and individuals. These references are included purely for informational purposes. The author does not endorse or have any affiliations with these entities, and any mention of specific names does not imply endorsement or recommendation. Readers are encouraged to conduct their own research and exercise independent judgment when considering any referenced sources.

By reading this book, you acknowledge and agree that you are solely responsible for your own health and dietary decisions.

# About This Book

**Plant-Based Nutrition for Beginners: The Essential Guide to Achieving Optimal Health Naturally with Constant Vegetable Consumption** serves as a crucial resource for those seeking to transform their health and well-being through the power of plant-based eating. This book not only introduces readers to the fundamental concepts of plant-based nutrition but also emphasizes the numerous health benefits associated with a diet rich in fruits and vegetables. By dispelling common myths and misconceptions, it empowers individuals to make informed dietary choices that align with their health goals.

One of the core strengths of this guide lies in its comprehensive exploration of plant-based nutrition, delving into the intricacies of dietary choices that promote overall health. Readers will gain a clear understanding of what constitutes a plant-based diet and the myriad advantages it offers, such as improved heart health, enhanced digestion, and increased energy levels. Moreover, the book highlights the environmental sustainability of plant-based eating, encouraging readers to consider the broader impact of their dietary choices on the planet. By acknowledging the diversity in plant-based eating styles, it fosters an inclusive atmosphere where individuals can find their unique path toward optimal health.

Getting started on a plant-based journey can be daunting, which is why the guide emphasizes the importance of cultivating a positive mindset and setting realistic goals. It offers practical strategies for transitioning to a plant-based lifestyle, focusing on the foundational principles that underpin a balanced diet. Readers will find valuable resources, including recommended books and websites, as well as tips for connecting with supportive communities that share similar dietary aspirations. This emphasis on community and support networks helps individuals navigate the challenges of changing their eating habits while feeling connected to others on the same journey.

The book further elaborates on the significance of whole foods, key nutrients, and the role of hydration in achieving a balanced plant-based diet. It equips readers with essential tools to make healthier food choices, understand food labels, and shop smartly on a budget. Additionally, the guide provides practical advice on meal prepping and incorporating a variety of colorful fruits and vegetables into daily meals, which is vital for maximizing nutritional intake and enjoying a diverse diet.

In its exploration of plant-based proteins, the book demystifies common concerns about protein intake while offering a plethora of options that include legumes, nuts, and whole grains. It provides insightful cooking tips and addresses the importance of complete amino acid profiles, ensuring that readers feel confident in meeting their protein needs without animal products. The emphasis on essential nutrients like B12, iron, calcium, and omega-3s further enhances the reader's understanding of nutritional balance, with practical strategies for supplementation and food sourcing included to alleviate potential deficiencies.

Cooking techniques and meal planning are also highlighted as essential components of successful plant-based eating. By introducing readers to effective kitchen tools and diverse cooking methods, the guide makes plant-based cooking accessible and enjoyable. It provides a structured approach to meal planning, emphasizing variety and creativity while incorporating leftovers and seasonal produce to minimize waste and maximize flavor.

Navigating social situations can be a significant hurdle for those adopting a plant-based diet. This guide provides thoughtful strategies for communicating dietary choices to friends and family, ensuring that individuals feel supported and understood. By sharing tips for dining out and hosting plant-based gatherings, it empowers readers to embrace their dietary preferences confidently while engaging with others.

Common concerns and FAQs are addressed comprehensively, offering reassurance to beginners who may be anxious about their new lifestyle. The guide emphasizes the importance of self-compassion and provides tools for overcoming challenges, making it clear that dietary transitions are a personal journey that can be navigated successfully with the right mindset and support.

Overall, **Plant-Based Nutrition for Beginners** serves as an essential roadmap for individuals eager to embark on a transformative journey toward better health and sustainability through plant-based eating. Its engaging and informative tone, coupled with practical guidance, makes it an invaluable resource for anyone seeking to thrive on a plant-based diet while celebrating the rich diversity of plant-based cuisine.

# Table of Contents

# Introduction

## What Does Plant-Based Nutrition Mean?

Plant-based nutrition focuses on foods derived primarily from plants. This includes fruits, vegetables, whole grains, nuts, seeds, and legumes, while minimizing or eliminating animal products. To adopt this lifestyle, start by incorporating a variety of plant foods into your meals. For instance, swap out meat for lentils or beans in your favorite dishes and explore new recipes that highlight seasonal vegetables.

Understanding that plant-based does not necessarily mean "vegan" or "vegetarian" is key. Many people adopt a plant-based approach by simply increasing their intake of plant foods while still enjoying some animal products. This can be achieved by designating certain days of the week as meatless, allowing for a gradual transition towards a more plant-focused diet.

# Health Benefits Associated with a Plant-Based Diet

Adopting a plant-based diet is linked to numerous health benefits, including improved heart health, weight management, and lower risks of chronic diseases such as diabetes and certain cancers. To experience these benefits, focus on consuming a variety of colorful fruits and vegetables daily. Aim for at least five servings of fruits and vegetables, and incorporate whole grains, legumes, and healthy fats like avocados and nuts.

Additionally, transitioning to a plant-based diet can enhance digestion due to the increased fiber intake from whole foods. This can be easily implemented by starting your day with a fiber-rich breakfast, such as oatmeal topped with berries and nuts, which helps sustain energy levels and promotes a healthy digestive system throughout the day.

# Common Misconceptions about Plant-Based Eating

One common misconception is that a plant-based diet lacks sufficient protein. In reality, many plant foods are rich in protein, such as lentils, chickpeas, quinoa, and tofu. Beginners should focus on incorporating these foods into meals, ensuring they meet their protein needs by combining different sources, like pairing rice with beans or adding nuts to salads.

Another misconception is that plant-based eating is overly restrictive and bland. However, plant-based diets can be incredibly diverse and flavorful. Experimenting with herbs, spices, and various cooking methods can enhance the taste of plant foods. For example, try roasting vegetables with olive oil and garlic or creating flavorful sauces using blended nuts or avocados to keep meals exciting.

# Environmental Impact of Plant-Based Diets

Plant-based diets are recognized for their positive impact on the environment, as they generally require fewer natural resources and produce lower greenhouse gas emissions compared to animal farming. To reduce your carbon footprint, consider meal prepping with seasonal and local produce, which is often fresher and requires less transportation.

Making small changes, like participating in a local community-supported agriculture (CSA) program or shopping at farmers' markets, can also support sustainable practices. When you consume seasonal fruits and vegetables, you contribute to a more sustainable food system while enjoying the benefits of fresh produce.

# Recognizing the Diversity in Plant-Based Eating Styles

Plant-based eating encompasses a wide range of styles, including vegetarian, vegan, flexitarian, and whole-foods plant-based diets. To find what works best for you, explore these different approaches and see how they fit into your lifestyle. For instance, if you love dairy, a lacto-vegetarian diet may be a good fit, allowing you to enjoy plant foods along with dairy products.

To simplify this exploration, create a weekly meal plan that incorporates various plant-based recipes aligned with your chosen style. This might include a mix of vegetarian meals, vegan days, or simply increasing the number of plant foods you consume daily. By keeping your meals diverse and exciting, you'll maintain motivation and enjoy the benefits of plant-based nutrition.

# Getting Started

## Cultivating a Positive Approach to Dietary Changes

Cultivating a positive mindset is crucial when making dietary changes. Begin by focusing on the benefits of a plant-based diet, such as increased energy, better digestion, and improved overall health. Instead of viewing this change as a restriction, embrace it as an opportunity to explore new foods and recipes. Celebrate small victories and stay open to experimenting with different fruits, vegetables, grains, and legumes, making the process enjoyable and fulfilling.

To reinforce this positive mindset, consider keeping a journal where you can record your feelings, progress, and new discoveries. Surround yourself with supportive communities, whether online or in-person, that encourage your journey. Engage with others who share similar goals and interests, and participate in discussions or workshops that promote a positive outlook on plant-based living. This supportive environment can significantly enhance your motivation and commitment.

## How to Set Realistic Health Goals

Setting realistic health goals is a fundamental step in adopting a plant-based diet. Start by identifying specific, measurable, achievable, relevant, and time-bound (SMART) goals that align with your lifestyle. For example, you might aim to incorporate at least one new plant-based meal into your weekly menu or reduce your meat consumption by one meal per week. Having clear and attainable goals helps you stay focused and motivated as you transition.

Once you've set your goals, create a plan of action that includes shopping lists, meal prep schedules, and resources for recipes. Regularly revisit your goals to assess your progress and make adjustments as needed. Celebrate your successes, no matter how small, and don't hesitate to revise your goals if you find they are too ambitious or not challenging enough. This flexible approach will help keep you engaged and motivated on your journey.

# Key Components of a Balanced Plant-Based Diet

Understanding the basic principles of a balanced plant-based diet is essential for success. Focus on incorporating a variety of whole foods, such as fruits, vegetables, whole grains, legumes, nuts, and seeds, to ensure you're getting all necessary nutrients. Each food group plays a vital role; for instance, fruits and vegetables provide essential vitamins and minerals, while whole grains and legumes offer fiber and protein.

To create balanced meals, aim for a colorful plate that includes foods from each of these categories. Plan your meals around seasonal produce and local options to enhance freshness and flavor. Don't forget to pay attention to protein sources, ensuring you include a variety of beans, lentils, tofu, and tempeh. By prioritizing diversity in your diet, you'll promote overall health and satisfaction while minimizing any nutritional deficiencies.

# CHAPTER 1:

# The Foundations of Plant-Based Nutrition

## Importance of Whole Foods over Processed Foods

Choosing whole foods over processed options is crucial for a healthy plant-based diet. Whole foods, such as fruits, vegetables, whole grains, nuts, and seeds, retain their natural nutrients and fiber. In contrast, processed foods often contain added sugars, unhealthy fats, and preservatives, which can detract from nutritional value and contribute to health issues. Incorporating more whole foods into your meals ensures that you're receiving a higher concentration of nutrients essential for optimal health.

To make the switch, start by filling your plate with whole foods during meals. Aim for at least half your plate to be filled with vegetables and fruits, along with whole grains like quinoa or brown rice. Avoid pre-packaged snacks and opt for whole food snacks like fresh fruits, nuts, or homemade energy bars. Over time, you'll notice improved energy levels and overall well-being as your body benefits from the wholesome nutrients.

## Key Nutrients to Focus On: Protein, Fiber, Vitamins, and Minerals

In a plant-based diet, focusing on key nutrients such as protein, fiber, vitamins, and minerals is vital for overall health. Plant-based protein sources include legumes, tofu, tempeh, and whole grains, providing essential amino acids. Fiber-rich foods, like fruits, vegetables, and whole grains, aid digestion and help maintain a healthy weight by keeping you feeling full longer.

To ensure you're getting adequate vitamins and minerals, incorporate a wide variety of colorful fruits and vegetables into your meals. Leafy greens, bell peppers, berries, and citrus fruits are excellent sources of vitamins A, C, and K. Consider keeping a food diary to track your nutrient intake, and consult a nutritionist if you have specific dietary concerns or restrictions.

## The Role of Fruits and Vegetables in a Balanced Diet

Fruits and vegetables are foundational to a balanced plant-based diet, providing essential nutrients, fiber, and antioxidants. They help reduce the risk of chronic diseases, support immune function, and promote overall well-being. Aim to fill half your plate with a variety of fruits and vegetables at every meal to maximize your nutrient intake.

To easily incorporate more fruits and vegetables, try adding them to smoothies, salads, and stir-fries. Keep fresh or frozen fruits and veggies on hand for quick snacks or meal additions. Experiment with new recipes that highlight these foods, and don't shy away from seasonal produce to enjoy the freshest flavors and nutrients.

## Understanding Macronutrients: Carbs, Fats, and Proteins

Macronutrients are the building blocks of your diet, consisting of carbohydrates, fats, and proteins. Each plays a crucial role in providing energy and supporting bodily functions. Carbohydrates, particularly from whole grains, fruits, and vegetables, should be the primary source of energy, while healthy fats from sources like avocados, nuts, and seeds provide essential fatty acids.

To maintain a balanced intake, aim for meals that include a source of each macronutrient. For example, a quinoa bowl with black beans (protein), avocado (healthy fat), and a variety of vegetables (carbs) creates a well-rounded meal. Being mindful of your macronutrient balance can enhance your energy levels and overall health.

# The Significance of Antioxidants and Photochemical

Antioxidants and photochemical are compounds found in plants that contribute to health by reducing inflammation and combating oxidative stress. These compounds are abundant in colorful fruits and vegetables, such as berries, kale, and sweet potatoes. Incorporating a variety of these foods can enhance your immune system and lower the risk of chronic diseases.

To boost your antioxidant intake, focus on consuming a rainbow of produce. Try adding berries to your breakfast, snacking on nuts, or creating vibrant salads with dark leafy greens, colorful peppers, and tomatoes. Consider herbs and spices like turmeric and ginger, which are also rich in beneficial photochemical.

## Hydration and Its Importance in a Plant-Based Diet

Staying hydrated is essential for overall health, particularly on a plant-based diet that emphasizes fiber-rich foods. Proper hydration aids digestion, nutrient absorption, and overall bodily functions. Aim to drink at least eight 8-ounce glasses of water daily, and increase your intake if you are physically active.

Incorporating hydrating foods like cucumbers, watermelon, and oranges can also boost your fluid intake. Consider starting your day with a glass of water and making it a habit to drink water before meals. Herbal teas and infused waters can provide variety and flavor while keeping you hydrated.

## Reading Food Labels for Healthier Choices

Understanding how to read food labels can help you make healthier choices in a plant-based diet. Look for products with minimal ingredients, and prioritize those without added sugars, unhealthy fats, or artificial additives. Pay attention to serving sizes and the percentage of daily values for key nutrients, ensuring that you're meeting your dietary needs.

When shopping, choose brands that emphasize whole ingredients and transparent labeling. If a product's label is difficult to understand or includes many unrecognizable ingredients, it might be better to opt for whole food alternatives. Familiarizing yourself with food labels can empower you to make informed decisions while grocery shopping.

## Tips for Grocery Shopping on a Budget

Grocery shopping on a budget is achievable with a bit of planning. Start by creating a weekly meal plan that outlines the meals you want to prepare, and make a corresponding shopping list. This approach helps avoid impulse purchases and ensures you buy only what you need for nutritious meals.

Consider shopping at local farmers' markets for fresh produce at lower prices, and take advantage of sales and discounts at grocery stores. Buying in bulk for grains, beans, and nuts can also save money. Preparing meals at home rather than purchasing pre-packaged foods will not only reduce costs but also enhance your cooking skills and ensure you know exactly what's in your meals.

## Meal Prepping for Success

Meal prepping is an effective strategy for maintaining a plant-based diet while saving time and effort during the week. Set aside a few hours on the weekend to prepare your meals, focusing on batch cooking grains, beans, and roasted vegetables. Store these in individual containers for easy access throughout the week.

To make meal prep successful, invest in good quality storage containers and label them with meal names and dates. Create a variety of meals using different combinations of grains, proteins, and vegetables to keep things interesting. By planning and preparing in advance, you're more likely to stick to your healthy eating goals.

# Incorporating a Variety of Colors in Your Diet

Eating a variety of colors in your diet ensures that you're getting a range of nutrients and health benefits. Each color in fruits and vegetables signifies different vitamins and minerals, so filling your plate with a rainbow can enhance your overall nutrition. Aim to include red, orange, yellow, green, blue, and purple foods in your meals.

To make this practical, try starting each meal with a colorful salad or smoothie. Experiment with different fruits and vegetables, such as adding blueberries to your oatmeal or roasted carrots to your dinner. By intentionally incorporating diverse colors, you'll not only improve your nutrient intake but also make your meals visually appealing.

# How to Transition Gradually to a Plant-Based Diet

Transitioning to a plant-based diet can be easier when done gradually. Start by incorporating more plant-based meals into your routine, perhaps by designating specific days as "meatless." Explore various plant-based recipes to discover new flavors and cooking methods, making the transition more enjoyable.

As you become comfortable, gradually replace animal-based products with plant-based alternatives, such as almond milk instead of dairy milk or lentils instead of meat. Listen to your body and adjust the transition pace according to your comfort level. With time, you'll find that embracing a plant-based lifestyle can be both satisfying and rewarding.

## The Significance of Portion Control

Understanding portion control is vital in a plant-based diet to ensure you're consuming the right amounts of food for your body's needs. Overeating, even healthy foods, can lead to weight gain and digestive discomfort.

Familiarize yourself with appropriate serving sizes for different food groups to better manage your intake.

To practice portion control, use smaller plates and bowls, which can help create the illusion of a fuller plate with less food. Also, pay attention to hunger cues and eat mindfully, allowing yourself to savor each bite. By being aware of portion sizes, you can enjoy a diverse range of foods while maintaining a balanced diet.

## Understanding Food Allergies and Intolerances

Being aware of food allergies and intolerances is crucial when adopting a plant-based diet. Some common allergens, such as soy, nuts, and gluten, can be present in many plant-based foods. If you have known allergies, read ingredient labels carefully and consider consulting with a healthcare provider or nutritionist.

To navigate this, focus on whole foods that are naturally free from common allergens, such as fruits, vegetables, and grains like rice or quinoa.

# CHAPTER 2:

# Building Balanced Meals

## Components of a Balanced Plant-Based Meal

A balanced plant-based meal should include a variety of food groups: vegetables, fruits, whole grains, legumes, nuts, and seeds. Aim for a colorful plate that incorporates these components to ensure a range of nutrients. For example, combine leafy greens (like spinach) with a whole grain (such as quinoa), a protein source (like chickpeas), and healthy fats (like avocado or nuts). This combination not only supports overall health but also enhances the meal's taste and texture.

To assemble a balanced meal, start by choosing a base, such as a grain or leafy green, and then layer in your favorite vegetables. Add a protein source—think beans, lentils, or tofu—and finish with a sprinkle of seeds or nuts for healthy fats. Don't forget to include a serving of fruit for natural sweetness and additional nutrients.

## Importance of Combining Food Groups for Nutrient Absorption

Combining different food groups enhances nutrient absorption in your body. For instance, pairing vitamin C-rich foods, like bell peppers or citrus fruits, with iron-rich foods, such as spinach or lentils, can significantly boost iron absorption. This is especially important on a plant-based diet, where iron sources are primarily non-heme, which is less easily absorbed than heme iron from animal products.

Additionally, incorporating healthy fats from sources like avocado or olive oil can help absorb fat-soluble vitamins (A, D, E, K) from your meals. Aim to create meals that include various food groups together to maximize the nutritional benefits of each component. This practice ensures you're getting the most out of the foods you eat.

# Quick Meal Ideas for Breakfast, Lunch, and Dinner

For a quick and nutritious breakfast, consider a smoothie made with spinach, banana, and almond milk, or overnight oats topped with berries and nuts. Both options are easy to prepare and can be customized with your favorite ingredients. Another idea is avocado toast on whole-grain bread, topped with tomato slices and a sprinkle of chia seeds for added nutrition.

For lunch and dinner, simple meals can include a grain bowl with brown rice, roasted vegetables, and a protein like tofu or tempeh. Stir-fries are also a fast option; just sauté seasonal veggies with garlic and ginger and serve over quinoa or noodles. Always keep pre-chopped vegetables and canned beans on hand to speed up your meal prep.

## Strategies for Creating a Meal Plan

Creating a meal plan starts with setting aside time each week to decide what meals you want to prepare. Make a list of recipes you'd like to try and then write down the ingredients needed. Consider planning meals that use similar ingredients to reduce waste and save money. This will help streamline your shopping and cooking process.

When you create your plan, include flexibility for spontaneous meals or snacks. It's also helpful to prep ingredients in advance, such as washing and chopping vegetables, cooking grains, or making dressings. This way, when it's time to cook, you can assemble meals quickly, making the process less daunting and more enjoyable.

## The Role of Snacks in a Healthy Diet

Snacks can play an essential role in maintaining energy levels and preventing overeating at meals. Opt for healthy, whole food snacks like fresh fruit, raw vegetables with hummus, or a handful of nuts. These options provide nutrients and help curb hunger between meals, keeping your energy stable throughout the day.

To make snacking easier, prepare snack bags or containers at the beginning of the week. Fill them with portioned amounts of nuts, cut-up vegetables, or whole-grain crackers. Having healthy snacks readily available can help you make better choices and avoid reaching for processed foods when hunger strikes.

## Understanding Serving Sizes for Different Food Groups

Understanding serving sizes is crucial for maintaining a balanced diet. Familiarize yourself with the recommended portions for different food groups—typically, a serving of grains is about one cup cooked, while a serving of vegetables is roughly one cup raw or half a cup cooked. Learning these measurements can help you better gauge how much you should be eating.

To visualize serving sizes, consider using your hand as a guide: one serving of protein is about the size of your palm, while a serving of healthy fats (like nut butter) should fit into your thumb. Keeping these guidelines in mind while preparing meals can help ensure you're eating appropriate amounts for a balanced plant-based diet.

# How to Use Herbs and Spices for Flavor Without Calories

Herbs and spices are fantastic tools for enhancing flavor in your meals without adding extra calories. Fresh herbs like basil, cilantro, and parsley can add brightness to salads, sauces, and soups. Dried spices such as cumin, paprika, and turmeric can deepen flavors in stews, curries, and roasted dishes.

Experimenting with different combinations of herbs and spices can transform a simple dish into something exciting. For instance, try adding garlic powder and smoked paprika to roasted vegetables, or use ginger and turmeric in stir-fries. This approach allows you to enjoy flavorful meals while keeping calories low, supporting your health goals.

## Incorporating Fermented Foods for Gut Health

Fermented foods are excellent for promoting gut health, as they contain beneficial probiotics. Common options include yogurt (look for plant-based varieties), sauerkraut, kimchi, and miso. Incorporating these foods into your diet can enhance digestion and support overall immune health.

To add fermented foods, try using them as toppings or sides. For example, add sauerkraut to a sandwich, toss some kimchi into a stir-fry, or use miso in soups or dressings. Start with small servings to see how your body reacts and gradually increase your intake for optimal gut health.

## Tips for Dining Out on a Plant-Based Diet

Dining out on a plant-based diet can be enjoyable with a little preparation. Before you go out, check the restaurant's menu online to see if they offer plant-based options. Many restaurants are accommodating and can modify dishes to suit your dietary preferences—don't hesitate to ask.

When ordering, focus on salads, grain bowls, or vegetable-based dishes. You can also request substitutions, such as replacing meat with extra veggies or beans. Always communicate your dietary needs to the staff to ensure your meal aligns with your plant-based goals.

## Adapting Recipes to Be Plant-Based

Adapting recipes to fit a plant-based lifestyle is easier than it might seem. Start by replacing animal products with plant-based alternatives: use almond milk instead of cow's milk, swap eggs for flaxseed or chia seed mixtures, and substitute meat with legumes, tofu, or tempeh. Many traditional recipes can be modified with simple ingredient changes.

Consider exploring plant-based cookbooks or blogs for inspiration and ideas. Look for recipes that highlight vegetables and grains, making it easier to experiment and discover new dishes. With practice, you'll find that converting favorite recipes into plant-based versions can be both fun and satisfying.

# Importance of Listening to Your Body's Hunger Cues

Listening to your body's hunger cues is essential for maintaining a healthy relationship with food. Pay attention to how you feel before and after meals; are you truly hungry, or are you eating out of boredom or stress? Recognizing these signals can help you make more mindful eating choices.

When you feel hungry, opt for nourishing foods that will satisfy your cravings. Give yourself permission to eat when you're hungry and stop when you're full. Practicing this awareness can lead to a more intuitive approach to eating, promoting better digestion and overall well-being.

## Sample Daily Meal Plans

A sample daily meal plan can help beginners visualize what a plant-based diet looks like in practice. For breakfast, consider oatmeal topped with fresh fruit and nuts. Lunch might include a quinoa salad with chickpeas, vegetables, and a light dressing, while dinner could feature a hearty vegetable stir-fry with brown rice. Snacks can be fresh fruit, raw vegetables with hummus, or a handful of mixed nuts.

Feel free to adjust the meal plan based on personal preferences and seasonal ingredients. Creating variety not only makes meals more enjoyable but also ensures a broader range of nutrients in your diet. Regularly rotating different recipes will keep your meals exciting and satisfying.

## Mindful Eating Practices

Mindful eating is about being present during meals, which enhances enjoyment and satisfaction. To practice this, minimize distractions—turn off the TV and put away your phone while eating. Take the time to appreciate the colors, textures, and flavors of your food, which can enhance your meal experience.

Another aspect of mindful eating is eating slowly and savoring each bite. Try to chew thoroughly and put down your fork between bites to fully engage with your meal.

# CHAPTER 3:

# Exploring Plant-Based Proteins

## Overview of Plant-Based Protein Sources

Plant-based protein sources are diverse and abundant, making it easier for beginners to incorporate them into their diets. Key sources include legumes (like lentils and chickpeas), nuts, seeds, whole grains, and soy products. Each category offers unique flavors and textures, allowing for creative meal preparation.

To get started, focus on incorporating a variety of these protein sources into your meals. For instance, try adding black beans to salads, sprinkling seeds on oatmeal, or incorporating quinoa into stir-fries. This approach not only enhances protein intake but also ensures you benefit from the range of nutrients these foods provide.

# Comparing Protein Content of Various Foods

Understanding the protein content in different foods can help you make informed dietary choices. For example, legumes typically provide about 15-20 grams of protein per cooked cup, while nuts and seeds offer around 5-7 grams per ounce. Whole grains like quinoa provide about 8 grams per cooked cup, whereas tofu can have as much as 20 grams per cup.

When planning meals, look for combinations that maximize protein content. A meal containing lentils and brown rice, for instance, offers a higher protein profile than either food alone. Use food labels and online resources to compare protein contents easily and choose foods that align with your nutritional goals.

## How to Combine Proteins for Complete Amino Acids

Combining different protein sources can ensure you obtain all essential amino acids. While most plant-based proteins are not complete (meaning they don't contain all nine essential amino acids), you can easily create complete proteins by pairing foods. For example, combine rice and beans, or hummus with whole-grain bread to achieve a balanced amino acid profile.

To simplify this process, plan meals that naturally combine these foods. A veggie burrito with black beans and brown rice or a peanut butter sandwich on whole-grain bread are both delicious and nutritionally complete. Keeping a list of complementary protein pairs can help make meal planning easier and more effective.

## The Role of Legumes, Nuts, and Seeds

Legumes, nuts, and seeds play a crucial role in a plant-based diet by providing not only protein but also fiber, healthy fats, and essential vitamins and minerals. Legumes like lentils, chickpeas, and black beans are excellent protein sources that can be easily added to soups, stews, and salads. Nuts and seeds add crunch and flavor to dishes while providing protein and healthy omega-3 fatty acids.

To incorporate these foods, consider adding a handful of nuts to your morning oatmeal or using legumes as the base for your main dish. For instance, making a chickpea salad or a lentil soup can boost your protein intake while also offering a variety of nutrients essential for overall health.

## Benefits of Whole Grains as Protein Sources

Whole grains are not only a source of carbohydrates but also provide a moderate amount of protein. Foods like quinoa, farro, and barley offer a unique nutritional profile, delivering fiber, vitamins, and minerals alongside their protein content. Incorporating whole grains into your meals can enhance satiety and provide lasting energy.

To reap the benefits, experiment with different whole grains in your diet. Substitute white rice with quinoa or brown rice, or use barley in salads or soups. This not only improves the nutritional value of your meals but also adds variety in taste and texture.

## Cooking Tips for Beans and Legumes

Cooking beans and legumes can be straightforward with a few simple techniques. Start by soaking dried beans overnight to reduce cooking time and improve digestibility. Rinse them well, then cook in fresh water, bringing them to a boil before simmering until tender. Canned beans can also be a quick alternative—just rinse them to remove excess sodium.

To enhance the flavor, consider seasoning beans during cooking with herbs, spices, or aromatics like onion and garlic. Using legumes in soups, stews, or salads not only boosts protein content but also adds creaminess and richness to your dishes.

# Understanding Soy Products: Tofu, Tempeh, and Edamame

Soy products are versatile and nutrient-dense options in plant-based diets. Tofu, which comes in various textures (soft, firm, extra-firm), can be used in savory dishes or sweet smoothies. Tempeh, a fermented soybean product, offers a nutty flavor and is excellent when marinated and grilled. Edamame, young soybeans, can be steamed and enjoyed as a snack or added to salads.

To incorporate these products, try stir-frying tofu with vegetables or making a tempeh sandwich. Adding edamame to your salads or grain bowls provides a protein boost and vibrant color to your meals.

# Protein Supplements: When and Why to Use Them

Protein supplements can be helpful for individuals who may struggle to meet their protein needs through food alone. Common forms include protein powders derived from pea, brown rice, or hemp. These supplements can easily be added to smoothies, oatmeal, or baked goods to increase protein intake without significantly changing your diet.

Before using protein supplements, assess your dietary habits to determine if you truly need them. If your meals already include a variety of protein sources, supplements may not be necessary. However, they can be beneficial for athletes or those with specific dietary restrictions looking to ensure adequate protein consumption.

## The Impact of Protein on Muscle Maintenance and Weight Loss

Protein plays a vital role in muscle maintenance and weight management. Consuming adequate protein helps preserve lean muscle mass during weight loss and supports recovery after exercise. Studies suggest that a higher protein intake can also enhance feelings of fullness, which may assist in reducing overall calorie intake.

To utilize protein for muscle maintenance, include a source of protein in every meal and snack. This could be as simple as pairing a piece of fruit with nut butter or adding a serving of beans to a salad. Consistency is key; ensure that you're incorporating protein-rich foods daily.

## Addressing Common Protein-Related Concerns

Common concerns about protein in plant-based diets often include adequate intake and amino acid completeness. However, as long as you consume a variety of protein sources throughout the day, you can easily meet your protein needs without animal products. Education on food choices can help dispel myths surrounding protein deficiencies.

For those new to plant-based eating, consider tracking your meals for a week to understand your protein intake better. Use apps or food journals to monitor what you consume, helping you identify any gaps and ensuring you include a diverse range of protein sources in your diet.

## How Much Protein Do You Really Need?

Protein needs vary based on factors like age, activity level, and overall health. A general guideline is to aim for 0.8 grams of protein per kilogram of body weight for the average adult. Active individuals or athletes may require more, around 1.2 to 2.0 grams per kilogram, depending on their training intensity and goals.

To calculate your specific needs, determine your weight in kilograms and multiply by the appropriate protein factor. This can help you set daily protein goals and make informed decisions about your food choices to ensure you meet these targets.

# The Myth of Protein Deficiency in Plant-Based Diets

Many people believe that plant-based diets lack sufficient protein, but research shows that with careful planning, this is rarely the case. As long as individuals consume a variety of plant foods, they can easily meet their protein requirements. Foods like lentils, quinoa, and nuts provide ample protein along with other nutrients essential for health.

To combat the myth, focus on educating yourself about plant protein sources and their protein content. Incorporate a wide range of these foods into your meals to dispel any concerns about protein deficiency, ensuring you enjoy a balanced and nutritious diet.

## Recipes for High-Protein Plant-Based Meals

Creating high-protein plant-based meals can be both simple and delicious. Consider recipes like a quinoa salad with black beans and avocado, a hearty lentil soup, or a chickpea curry with brown rice. These meals not only provide ample protein but also deliver a variety of flavors and textures.

When trying out recipes, aim for dishes that combine different protein sources to maximize your intake. For example, making a stir-fry with tofu and mixed vegetables served over quinoa can be a nutritious and satisfying way to meet your protein goals while enjoying a tasty meal.

# CHAPTER 4:

# Essential Nutrients in a Plant-Based Diet

## Key Nutrients That May Require Attention: B12, Iron, Calcium, Omega-3s

When transitioning to a plant-based diet, it's crucial to be mindful of specific nutrients that may be less abundant in plant foods. Vitamin B12, primarily found in animal products, is essential for nerve function and blood formation, while iron, calcium, and omega-3 fatty acids also require attention. A deficiency in any of these nutrients can lead to health issues, so understanding their sources and importance is key for beginners.

To ensure adequate intake, consider fortified foods or supplements, particularly for B12 and omega-3s, which are often less available in plant-based diets. Additionally, it's helpful to incorporate a variety of foods rich in these nutrients to support overall health and well-being.

## Food Sources Rich in These Essential Nutrients

To maintain a balanced plant-based diet, incorporate foods that are high in essential nutrients. For Vitamin B12, fortified plant milks, nutritional yeast, and some breakfast cereals can provide necessary levels. Iron can be found in legumes, tofu, spinach, and quinoa, while calcium is abundant in fortified plant milks, leafy greens, and almonds. Omega-3s can be sourced from flaxseeds, chia seeds, and walnuts.

Including a diverse range of foods ensures you're not only meeting your nutritional needs but also enjoying a variety of flavors and textures. Meal planning around these foods can simplify your dietary choices and help maintain balance.

# Importance of Supplementation for Certain Vitamins

Supplementation can play a significant role in achieving optimal health on a plant-based diet. For example, Vitamin B12 supplementation is often recommended, as plant sources typically provide insufficient amounts. Similarly, Vitamin D may require supplementation, especially in regions with limited sunlight exposure, which is necessary for natural synthesis.

It's essential to consult with a healthcare professional before starting any supplements to determine individual needs and appropriate dosages. Regularly assessing your nutrient levels can also help guide supplementation strategies, ensuring you achieve optimal health without deficiencies.

# Signs and Symptoms of Nutrient Deficiencies

Being aware of the signs and symptoms of nutrient deficiencies can help you adjust your diet proactively.

Common indicators of B12 deficiency include fatigue, weakness, and neurological issues like numbness. For iron deficiency, symptoms often include dizziness, pale skin, and shortness of breath, while calcium deficiency may lead to muscle cramps and brittle bones.

Monitoring your body's signals and getting regular blood tests can help you stay informed about your nutrient status. If you notice persistent symptoms, it's crucial to evaluate your dietary habits and consider professional guidance to address any deficiencies.

## Balancing Nutrient Intake Through Food Choices

Achieving balance in your nutrient intake requires careful food choices. Aiming for a variety of whole foods such as fruits, vegetables, whole grains, nuts, and legumes will provide a spectrum of nutrients essential for health. Meal diversity not only enhances taste but also ensures you meet your nutritional needs more effectively.

One practical strategy is to use a "rainbow plate" concept, ensuring you include a range of colors in your meals. Each color often represents different nutrients, so this approach can naturally lead to a well-rounded nutrient intake.

## Tips for Improving Iron Absorption

Iron absorption can be enhanced through certain dietary practices. Combining iron-rich plant foods, such as beans and lentils, with Vitamin C sources, like citrus fruits or bell peppers, can significantly boost absorption. Additionally, cooking in cast iron pots can add iron to your food, further supporting your intake.

Avoiding coffee and tea during meals is also advisable, as tannins can inhibit iron absorption. By strategically planning your meals, you can ensure better utilization of iron from plant-based sources.

# Importance of Vitamin D and Sunlight Exposure

Vitamin D is vital for bone health and immune function, and it can be synthesized by the body through sunlight exposure. However, many people, especially those living in northern climates or with limited sun exposure, may require dietary sources or supplements. Foods such as fortified plant milks and mushrooms exposed to UV light can help meet your needs.

To maximize Vitamin D synthesis, aim to get about 15-30 minutes of sunlight several times a week, depending on your skin type and local climate. If sunlight is limited, discuss supplementation options with a healthcare provider to ensure adequate levels.

## Exploring Fortified Foods and Their Benefits

Fortified foods are an excellent option for beginners looking to enhance their nutrient intake without extensive meal planning. Products such as fortified plant milks, cereals, and nutritional yeast can provide essential vitamins and minerals that may be lacking in a strictly plant-based diet. This makes it easier to meet your nutritional needs with minimal effort.

When selecting fortified foods, always check labels for added nutrients and opt for products that align with your dietary goals. Incorporating these foods into your regular meals can simplify the process of maintaining a balanced diet.

## Understanding the Role of Fatty Acids

Fatty acids, particularly omega-3 and omega-6, are crucial for brain health and reducing inflammation. In a plant-based diet, it's essential to focus on sources of ALA (alpha-linolenic acid), a type of omega-3 found in flaxseeds, chia seeds, and walnuts. Balancing your intake of omega-6 fatty acids, typically found in vegetable oils, is also important to maintain a healthy ratio.

To ensure adequate omega-3 intake, incorporate ground flaxseed or chia seeds into smoothies, oatmeal, or baked goods. Regularly including these foods in your diet can help you achieve the right balance of fatty acids for optimal health.

## How to Track Nutrient Intake

Tracking your nutrient intake can provide valuable insights into your diet and help you make necessary adjustments. Many mobile apps are available that allow you to log your meals and analyze nutrient content easily. This practice can help you identify any deficiencies or excesses in your diet, guiding you toward a more balanced approach.

Start by noting the foods you typically consume and look for patterns in your nutrient intake. Regular tracking can help you stay accountable and make informed choices about food selection, ensuring you meet your health goals.

# Consulting with a Nutritionist for Personalized Guidance

Consulting a nutritionist can provide personalized insights and support as you transition to a plant-based diet. A nutritionist can help you develop a tailored meal plan that meets your specific needs, taking into account factors such as lifestyle, activity level, and health goals. Their expertise can help you navigate nutrient requirements and ensure you're making informed choices.

Schedule a consultation to discuss your dietary preferences and health concerns. With their guidance, you can establish a sustainable plant-based eating plan that promotes optimal health.

## Strategies for Maintaining Nutrient Balance

To maintain nutrient balance on a plant-based diet, implement strategies that promote diversity and nutrient density in your meals. Consider batch cooking meals that incorporate a variety of foods, which can save time while ensuring you consume a range of nutrients. Experimenting with new recipes can also keep your meals exciting and nutritious.

Another effective strategy is to create a weekly meal plan that includes nutrient-rich foods across all food groups. This can help you stay organized and ensure that you're not neglecting any essential nutrients throughout the week.

## Common Myths about Nutrients in Plant-Based Diets

Addressing common myths about plant-based nutrients can empower beginners to embrace this lifestyle confidently. A prevalent myth is that plant-based diets lack sufficient protein; however, many plant foods such as legumes, tofu, and quinoa are excellent protein sources. Another misconception is that it's challenging to meet vitamin and mineral needs; with proper planning and knowledge of food sources, it's entirely feasible.

Educating yourself about these myths can help you navigate the challenges of transitioning to a plant-based diet. By understanding the reality of nutrient availability, you can make informed choices and enjoy a well-rounded, healthy diet.

# CHAPTER 5:

# Cooking Techniques for Plant-Based Meals

## Essential Kitchen Tools and Equipment for Plant-Based Cooking

To embark on your plant-based cooking journey, equip your kitchen with essential tools. A good set of knives, cutting boards, and measuring cups are crucial for precision in preparation. Invest in quality cookware such as non-stick pans, a heavy-bottomed pot for soups and stews, and a high-speed blender for smoothies and sauces. Consider adding a food processor for tasks like chopping vegetables and making dips, which can save you time and effort.

In addition to basic utensils, specialty items like a spiralizer for vegetable noodles or a dehydrator for snacks can enhance your cooking experience. Don't forget storage containers for leftovers and meal prep, ideally glass or BPA-free plastic for safety and longevity.

Organizing your tools will streamline your cooking process and inspire creativity in the kitchen.

## Basic Cooking Methods: Steaming, Roasting, Sautéing, and More

Understanding basic cooking methods is key to creating delicious plant-based meals. Steaming vegetables preserves nutrients and enhances flavors, making it an ideal method for greens like broccoli or spinach. To steam, use a pot with a steaming basket or an electric steamer, ensuring the water doesn't touch the vegetables for optimal results.

Roasting brings out the natural sweetness of vegetables like carrots and sweet potatoes. Simply toss your chosen veggies with olive oil, salt, and your favorite spices, then spread them on a baking sheet and roast in a preheated oven at 400°F (200°C) until tender. Sautéing is another quick method; heat a small amount of oil in a skillet and cook chopped vegetables over medium-high heat until they're crisp-tender. Experiment with different combinations to find your favorites!

# Tips for Meal Prep and Batch Cooking

Meal prepping is a game-changer for maintaining a plant-based diet. Start by planning your meals for the week, making a shopping list that includes fresh produce, whole grains, legumes, and nuts. Set aside a few hours on the weekend to wash, chop, and portion out ingredients, which will make cooking during the week much faster and easier.

Batch cooking is another effective strategy. Prepare large quantities of grains, beans, and roasted vegetables that can be stored in the refrigerator or freezer for quick meals. Label your containers with dates to keep track of freshness, and mix and match these prepped items throughout the week to create varied meals without the daily hassle of cooking from scratch.

# How to Use a Slow Cooker for Easy Meals

A slow cooker can simplify your plant-based cooking by allowing you to prepare meals with minimal effort. Start by adding your desired ingredients—like chopped vegetables, grains, and broth—into the slow cooker. Set it on low for 6-8 hours or high for 3-4 hours, depending on your schedule.

Experiment with soups, stews, or grain dishes like quinoa or brown rice. The slow cooker not only tenderizes vegetables but also melds flavors beautifully. For added convenience, you can set it up in the morning before heading out, ensuring a warm, delicious meal awaits you when you return home.

## Exploring Different Cuisines and Their Plant-Based Options

Diving into global cuisines can provide a wealth of plant-based inspiration. Start by researching cuisines known for their vegetable-forward dishes, like

Mediterranean, Indian, or Thai. Many traditional recipes can be easily adapted to be plant-based; for example, use chickpeas in place of meat in curries or make a lentil shepherd's pie.

Explore local markets to find unique spices and ingredients that can elevate your dishes. Try incorporating staples like lentils, beans, and whole grains to diversify your meals. Don't hesitate to experiment with flavors and techniques, as this will not only enhance your culinary skills but also make your plant-based diet more enjoyable.

## How to Adapt Traditional Recipes for a Plant-Based Diet

Adapting traditional recipes to fit a plant-based diet is a great way to maintain your favorite meals while embracing healthier choices. Start by identifying the key ingredients in your favorite recipes, such as meat, dairy, or eggs, and find suitable plant-based substitutes. For instance, use plant-based milks like almond or soy instead of cow's milk, and try silken tofu or flaxseed meal as an egg replacement in baking.

Modify cooking times and methods as needed to ensure your plant-based adaptations maintain their original texture and flavor. It's essential to taste as you go, adjusting spices and seasonings to achieve the desired taste. This process encourages creativity in the kitchen and allows you to keep enjoying the foods you love.

## Understanding Food Storage and Preservation Techniques

Proper food storage and preservation techniques are vital for minimizing waste and maximizing the freshness of your plant-based ingredients. Begin by learning how to store fruits and vegetables correctly; for instance, keep potatoes in a cool, dark place and store leafy greens wrapped in damp paper towels to maintain moisture.

Explore preservation methods like freezing, canning, and fermenting to extend the life of your produce. Freezing is particularly effective for fruits and vegetables, as it locks in nutrients and flavor. If you're interested in fermentation, consider starting with simple recipes like pickles or sauerkraut, which add probiotics to your diet and enhance the taste of many dishes.

## Incorporating Raw Foods into Your Diet

Adding raw foods to your diet is a great way to boost nutrient intake and introduce a variety of flavors and textures. Start by incorporating raw fruits and vegetables into your meals; think salads, smoothies, or snacks like carrot sticks with hummus. Experiment with raw recipes such as zoodles (zucchini noodles) or raw desserts made from blended nuts and dates.

Consider trying raw food days or meals to help your body adapt gradually. Listen to your body and find the right balance between raw and cooked foods that works for you. This variety not only enriches your diet but also helps in discovering new ways to enjoy plant-based eating.

# Creative Ways to Use Leftovers

Transforming leftovers into new meals can help reduce food waste while keeping your diet interesting. Start by storing leftovers in clear containers, so they're visible and easily accessible. Use them as the base for new dishes, like turning roasted vegetables into a hearty grain bowl topped with a flavorful sauce or combining them with fresh greens to make a vibrant salad.

Think outside the box by creating soups or stir-fries from assorted leftovers. For example, blend leftover vegetables into a smooth soup or sauté them with tofu and your favorite sauce for a quick stir-fry. Not only does this save time and money, but it also encourages creativity in your cooking.

## Importance of Seasonal Cooking

Cooking with seasonal ingredients can enhance the freshness and flavor of your meals. Start by familiarizing yourself with what fruits and vegetables are in season in your area, as these ingredients are typically at their peak flavor and nutritional value. Use local farmers' markets as a resource for sourcing fresh produce while supporting your community.

Incorporating seasonal cooking into your meal planning not only benefits your health but also helps reduce your carbon footprint by lowering the demand for out-of-season produce. Create a seasonal recipe book to help inspire your meals throughout the year and experiment with new ingredients as they come into season.

## Using Online Resources for Plant-Based Recipes

The internet is a treasure trove of resources for plant-based cooking. Explore websites, blogs, and social media platforms dedicated to plant-based diets. Look for recipe sites that allow you to filter by dietary preferences and ingredients, making it easy to find meals that fit your needs.

YouTube is also a great platform for learning cooking techniques and discovering new recipes through visual guidance. Consider joining online communities or forums where you can share experiences, ask questions, and exchange tips with others on a similar plant-based journey.

## Cooking for Families and Accommodating Diverse Preferences

Cooking for families requires creativity and flexibility, especially when accommodating diverse preferences. Start by planning meals that can be customized, such as tacos or grain bowls, allowing family members to choose their toppings. This approach promotes inclusivity while ensuring everyone gets to enjoy the meal.

Engage your family in the cooking process, encouraging them to help with meal prep or select recipes. This not only makes mealtime more enjoyable but also fosters a sense of togetherness. Be open to experimenting with new flavors and dishes that cater to different tastes, creating a positive and collaborative cooking environment.

# Simple and Quick Recipes for Busy Individuals

For those with hectic schedules, simple and quick recipes are essential to maintaining a plant-based diet. Focus on meals that require minimal ingredients and can be prepared in under 30 minutes. Examples include stir-frying frozen vegetables with pre-cooked quinoa or making a quick salad with canned beans, fresh greens, and a homemade dressing.

Utilize tools like pressure cookers or microwaves to speed up cooking times. Batch-cook grains and legumes ahead of time, so you can easily throw together meals on busy days. Having a few go-to recipes that are nutritious and satisfying can help you stay committed to your plant-based lifestyle, even when time is tight.

# CHAPTER 6:

# Meal Planning and Preparation

## The Benefits of Meal Planning for Plant-Based Diets

Meal planning simplifies your weekly cooking routine, allowing you to have a clear vision of what you'll eat each day. This approach not only helps in reducing food waste but also ensures you incorporate a variety of vegetables and nutrients into your diet. By planning your meals, you can create balanced dishes that cater to your dietary needs while avoiding impulse purchases that often lead to unhealthy choices.

Additionally, meal planning saves time and stress. With a set plan, you can prepare ingredients in advance, making it easier to whip up healthy meals quickly. Knowing what meals are on the agenda can help streamline grocery shopping, ensuring you only buy what you need. This foresight can lead to better nutritional choices and overall improved health.

# Step-by-Step Guide to Creating a Weekly Meal Plan

Begin your weekly meal planning by assessing your schedule for the week. Consider your commitments and how many meals you'll need to prepare at home. Once you know your availability, choose a variety of recipes that include different vegetables, grains, proteins, and healthy fats to ensure a balanced diet. Aim for at least three meals for each day, incorporating diverse ingredients to keep things interesting.

Next, write down your meals for each day on a calendar or planner. This visual aid helps you see what you will cook and eat. Once your meals are planned, make a grocery list based on the ingredients required for each recipe. This list not only makes shopping easier but also helps you avoid buying unnecessary items, keeping your plant-based diet focused and affordable.

# How to Organize Your Grocery List Effectively

To organize your grocery list, first categorize your items based on the layout of your grocery store. Common categories include produce, grains, canned goods, dairy alternatives, and snacks. By grouping similar items together, you can navigate the store more efficiently, saving time and ensuring you don't forget any essentials.

Consider using a digital app or a note-taking tool on your phone to create and manage your grocery list. Many apps allow you to check off items as you shop, helping you stay organized. Regularly updating your list based on your meal plans will not only keep your pantry stocked with healthy options but also prevent the temptation to buy processed or unhealthy foods.

# Tips for Batch Cooking and Freezing Meals

Batch cooking involves preparing large quantities of meals at once, making it a great time-saver for a plant-based diet. Start by selecting a few recipes that freeze well, such as soups, stews, or grain bowls. Cook the meals on a day when you have extra time, like the weekend, and portion them into individual servings for easy reheating later in the week.

When freezing meals, use airtight containers or freezer bags to prevent freezer burn. Label each container with the date and contents for easy identification. By having ready-to-eat meals in your freezer, you can ensure that healthy, plant-based options are always available, even on the busiest of days.

# Importance of Variety in Your Meal Plan

Incorporating a variety of foods into your meal plan is essential for obtaining a wide range of nutrients. Aim to include different vegetables, legumes, grains, and proteins throughout the week. This not only keeps meals exciting but also helps you discover new flavors and textures that can enhance your eating experience.

To achieve variety, try choosing a "theme" for each day or meal, such as Italian, Mexican, or Asian cuisines. Experimenting with different spices and cooking techniques can also help in keeping your meals diverse. This creativity can turn a simple vegetable into a delicious dish, making it easier to maintain your plant-based lifestyle.

## Adapting Meal Plans to Different Seasons

Seasonal eating involves adjusting your meal plans based on the availability of fresh produce. In spring and summer, focus on lighter dishes featuring fresh fruits and leafy greens, while in fall and winter, incorporate heartier vegetables like squash and root vegetables. This approach not only ensures your meals are flavorful but also supports local agriculture and reduces your carbon footprint.

To adapt your meal plans, start by visiting local farmers' markets or checking grocery stores for seasonal produce. Plan your meals around these items, incorporating them into your recipes. This practice enhances the taste of your meals and keeps your diet varied and aligned with what is naturally available throughout the year.

## How to Incorporate Leftovers Creatively

Leftovers are a great opportunity to reduce food waste while saving time on meal prep. Get creative by transforming leftovers into new dishes. For instance, leftover roasted vegetables can be added to a grain bowl or blended into a soup, while unused grains can serve as a base for a stir-fry.

To make this process easier, designate a specific day for "leftover creations," where you use up what's in your fridge. This can also encourage you to experiment with flavors and textures, helping you learn to cook on the fly and find unique combinations that you enjoy.

## Planning for Snacks and Treats

Snacks play a crucial role in maintaining energy levels throughout the day, especially on a plant-based diet. Plan for healthy snacks by preparing a selection in advance, such as chopped vegetables with hummus, fruit smoothies, or homemade energy bars. Having these snacks ready ensures you won't resort to unhealthy options when hunger strikes.

Incorporate a balance of nutrients in your snacks, including proteins, healthy fats, and complex carbohydrates. This balance will keep you satisfied longer and support overall health. Consider packing snacks in portable containers, making it easier to grab-and-go whether you're at work, school, or on the move.

## Using Technology for Meal Planning

Utilizing technology can streamline your meal planning process significantly. Various apps and websites allow you to plan meals, create grocery lists, and even track your nutritional intake. Many of these platforms provide recipe suggestions based on dietary preferences, helping you discover new plant-based meals to try.

Additionally, consider using meal prep videos or online cooking classes that demonstrate plant-based cooking techniques. This resource can boost your confidence in the kitchen and introduce you to a variety of cooking styles and ingredient combinations, making the meal preparation process more enjoyable and efficient.

## How to Adjust Plans for Special Occasions

When preparing for special occasions, consider how to adapt your plant-based meal plan to accommodate guests or celebrations. Start by selecting recipes that can easily be scaled up to serve larger groups, such as a big vegetable lasagna or a hearty salad. Having a few crowd-pleasing recipes on hand can help you feel prepared for any event.

Don't hesitate to experiment with festive ingredients and flavors that match the occasion. You can incorporate seasonal produce or traditional dishes with a plant-based twist. By planning ahead, you can enjoy celebrations while staying true to your dietary goals without feeling overwhelmed.

## Tips for Dining Out and Traveling While Maintaining a Plant-Based Diet

When dining out, look for restaurants that cater to plant-based diets or offer customizable options. Many places now feature vegetarian or vegan dishes, and you can often ask for modifications to suit your preferences. Familiarizing yourself with the menu in advance can help you make healthier choices and feel confident ordering.

Traveling can be more challenging, but preparation is key. Research restaurants and grocery stores at your destination ahead of time. Packing snacks like nuts, granola bars, or dried fruit can also keep you fueled and prevent unhealthy eating on the go. With a little planning, you can maintain your plant-based lifestyle while enjoying new experiences.

## Building a Personal Recipe Book

Creating a personal recipe book is a fun and rewarding way to organize your favorite plant-based dishes. Start by collecting recipes from various sources—cookbooks, online blogs, or family traditions. You can use a binder, digital app, or even a blog to compile your recipes, ensuring easy access for future meal planning.

Include notes or modifications you've made to the recipes, allowing you to personalize each dish. This practice not only helps you remember how you made a dish but also encourages you to continue experimenting and improving your cooking skills as you refine your collection over time.

## Reflecting on and Adjusting Meal Plans as Needed

Regularly reflecting on your meal plans is crucial for adapting to your preferences and nutritional needs. At the end of each week, take a moment to evaluate what worked and what didn't. Did you enjoy the meals you prepared? Were there recipes you didn't like or found too time-consuming? Taking notes can help you refine your future meal plans.

Adjusting your meal plans based on these reflections is a key step in maintaining a sustainable plant-based diet. If certain meals are consistently left uneaten, consider replacing them with alternatives you know you'll enjoy. This ongoing evaluation and adjustment can lead to a more satisfying and effective approach to plant-based eating.

# CHAPTER 7:

# Navigating Social Situations

## Strategies for Discussing Your Diet with Friends and Family

When discussing your plant-based diet with friends and family, approach the conversation with positivity and openness. Start by sharing the reasons behind your dietary choices, whether it's for health, environmental, or ethical reasons. Engaging them with personal stories about the benefits you've experienced can create a more relatable dialogue. Offer to share recipes or cooking tips to spark their interest in plant-based meals, making it a collaborative discussion rather than a debate.

Be prepared for questions and differing opinions. Practice active listening and remain respectful of their views while standing firm in your choices. If they express concern or confusion, gently provide information or suggest resources for further reading.

This can help demystify your diet and foster a supportive environment for continued conversation.

## Tips for Attending Social Gatherings and Parties

Attending social gatherings while adhering to a plant-based diet can be enjoyable with a bit of preparation. Before the event, consider bringing a dish to share, ensuring there's at least one option that aligns with your dietary choices. This not only guarantees you'll have something to eat but also introduces others to delicious plant-based cuisine. Communicate with the host in advance to see if they can accommodate your dietary needs or if they'd like you to contribute a dish.

During the event, don't hesitate to explore the food options available. Many dishes can be modified or combined to create a plant-based meal. For example, salads can often be enhanced by asking for dressings on the side, or you might be able to skip cheese in pasta dishes. Remember to enjoy the social aspect of the gathering—focus on engaging with people rather than solely on food.

## How to Handle Criticism and Skepticism about Your Choices

Criticism about your plant-based choices can be challenging but can also serve as an opportunity to educate others. When confronted with skepticism, respond calmly and provide factual information to support your diet. Share your positive experiences and health improvements to illustrate the benefits, which can sometimes change minds more effectively than arguments. Maintain a non-defensive tone; it's essential to express your passion for your diet without appearing confrontational.

Additionally, be open to constructive criticism. Use it as a chance to engage in dialogue, addressing concerns without dismissing them outright. This not only helps you clarify your own beliefs but can also encourage a more supportive understanding among those around you.

# Finding Plant-Based Options at Restaurants

Finding plant-based options at restaurants starts with doing your homework. Before going out, check the menu online or call the restaurant to inquire about vegetarian and vegan offerings. Many places now have plant-based items, but knowing what to expect can save time and reduce stress. When at the restaurant, don't hesitate to customize your order; asking for substitutions like removing cheese or swapping out meat for extra vegetables can often yield satisfying meals.

If you're dining with others, suggest places known for their plant-based options. This can help ease any discomfort and allow everyone to enjoy the experience. Remember, your choice of dining establishment doesn't just support your diet; it can also introduce your friends to delicious plant-based cuisine.

# How to Host a Plant-Based Dinner Party

Hosting a plant-based dinner party can be a delightful way to share your dietary choices with others. Start by planning a diverse menu that showcases a variety of flavors and textures, such as appetizers, main dishes, and desserts. Use seasonal ingredients to ensure freshness and visual appeal. Prepare a dish that you feel confident making, and consider including a few crowd-pleasers, such as vegan tacos or a hearty vegetable lasagna.

Communicate clearly with your guests about the menu, allowing them to ask questions or express dietary restrictions. Providing a printed menu or recipe cards can add an engaging touch to the evening. Encourage interaction by involving your guests in the cooking process or serving family-style meals, which creates a communal atmosphere and highlights the enjoyment of plant-based eating.

# Communicating Dietary Restrictions Effectively

Effectively communicating dietary restrictions requires clarity and confidence. When sharing your plant-based preferences, be specific about what you do and do not eat. This helps others understand how they can accommodate your needs, whether in social settings or meal planning. Use simple language to explain your choices, and don't hesitate to share how these restrictions contribute to your health or well-being.

In group settings, proactively discuss your dietary restrictions before meal preparation. This ensures everyone is on the same page and can help brainstorm plant-based options that everyone can enjoy. Being clear and open about your needs fosters an inclusive environment that respects everyone's dietary choices.

# Tips for Traveling While Maintaining Your Diet

Traveling on a plant-based diet can be manageable with a little foresight. Before you embark on your journey, research local restaurants, markets, and grocery stores at your destination that cater to plant-based eaters. Apps and websites dedicated to vegan and vegetarian options can be extremely helpful. Packing snacks like nuts, fruit, or energy bars can also keep you fueled during long travels, especially when plant-based options might be limited.

When dining out while traveling, don't hesitate to ask about plant-based modifications or specific ingredients in dishes. Many chefs are willing to accommodate dietary preferences. In addition, consider staying in accommodations with kitchen facilities, allowing you to prepare simple meals with local ingredients, ensuring you stay on track with your dietary goals.

# How to Support Friends and Family in Their Dietary Changes

Supporting friends and family who want to adopt a plant-based diet involves encouragement and practical assistance. Start by listening to their motivations and concerns; understanding their reasons helps you provide tailored advice. Share recipes, meal plans, or even cook together to make the transition more enjoyable. Celebrating small victories and milestones along their journey reinforces their commitment and can strengthen your relationship.

Offer to join them in trying new foods or exploring plant-based restaurants together. This shared experience can alleviate any feelings of isolation they might feel while making changes. Additionally, provide resources like books or documentaries that inspired you, which can further motivate and educate them about the benefits of a plant-based lifestyle.

# Navigating Workplace Food Environments

Navigating food environments at work can present challenges but also opportunities to advocate for your plant-based diet. Start by preparing your meals and snacks to bring to work, ensuring you have healthy options available. If there are company events, offer to bring a plant-based dish that can be shared, allowing others to see how delicious and satisfying plant-based eating can be.

When colleagues bring in food, don't shy away from asking about ingredients. This promotes awareness and may encourage others to think about their food choices. Additionally, engage your coworkers in conversations about nutrition; this can create an open dialogue and may inspire them to explore plant-based options themselves.

# Importance of Being Flexible and Open-Minded

Flexibility and open-mindedness are crucial when adopting a plant-based diet. While it's essential to stay true to your dietary choices, allowing room for occasional indulgences or modifications can prevent feelings of deprivation and enhance your overall experience. Experimenting with different recipes and foods can lead to exciting culinary discoveries that keep your meals enjoyable and satisfying.

Being open-minded also extends to social situations. Embrace the possibility of trying plant-based dishes prepared by others, even if they differ from your typical preferences. This not only shows appreciation for their efforts but also helps expand your palate and fosters a sense of community around food.

# Engaging with Plant-Based Communities

Engaging with plant-based communities can provide support, inspiration, and a wealth of resources. Look for local groups, clubs, or online forums where you can share experiences, recipes, and tips with like-minded individuals. Attending meetups, workshops, or cooking classes can create connections and enrich your understanding of plant-based living.

Social media platforms are also valuable tools for engaging with plant-based communities. Follow influencers, chefs, or nutritionists who share insights, recipes, and encouragement. Participate in discussions or challenges that promote plant-based eating, making your journey more interactive and enjoyable.

## The Role of Social Media in Support and Inspiration

Social media can be a powerful ally in your plant-based journey, offering inspiration and support from a diverse community. Follow accounts that align with your dietary goals, such as those focusing on healthy recipes, meal prep tips, or motivational stories. Engage with content by liking, sharing, and commenting, which can create connections and foster a sense of belonging within the plant-based community.

Additionally, consider sharing your own experiences on social media. Document your meals, recipes, or tips for maintaining a plant-based lifestyle, which can inspire others and encourage dialogue. This reciprocal exchange of knowledge and encouragement not only strengthens your commitment but also helps others on their journey.

## Celebrating Milestones and Successes with Others

Celebrating milestones in your plant-based journey can be a motivating experience. Whether it's your first month of adhering to your diet or mastering a challenging recipe, acknowledge these achievements with friends or family. Share your success stories through gatherings, social media, or simply in conversations. This not only reinforces your commitment but also encourages others to support and join you in your endeavors.

Organizing small celebrations, like a potluck or a themed dinner night, can bring your community together and showcase your favorite plant-based dishes. Engaging in these shared experiences cultivates a positive atmosphere around your dietary choices and strengthens connections with those who support your lifestyle.

# CHAPTER 8:

# Common Concerns and FAQs

## Addressing Common Myths about Plant-Based Diets

Many myths surround plant-based diets, leading to misconceptions about their nutritional adequacy. One common myth is that plant-based diets lack protein. In reality, numerous plant sources—like lentils, beans, quinoa, and nuts—provide ample protein. Incorporating a variety of these foods into your meals ensures you receive sufficient protein without the need for animal products.

Another myth is that plant-based diets are bland or unappealing. In fact, a plant-based diet offers a vibrant array of flavors and textures. By exploring various cooking techniques, such as grilling, roasting, and stir-frying, you can create exciting dishes that are both satisfying and delicious, proving that plant-based eating can be as flavorful as any other diet.

# Understanding Potential Challenges: Cravings, Social Pressures, etc.

Transitioning to a plant-based diet can bring challenges, such as cravings for familiar foods or dealing with social pressures when dining out. Recognizing that cravings are natural can help you navigate them more effectively. Instead of resisting, try to find plant-based alternatives that satisfy those cravings, such as swapping cheese for cashew cheese or enjoying vegan desserts made from whole ingredients.

Social situations can also pose challenges, especially if friends or family do not share your dietary preferences. To mitigate this, communicate your dietary choices openly with your social circle and suggest plant-based options when hosting gatherings. Being proactive can help you feel more comfortable in social settings and encourage others to explore plant-based eating as well.

# FAQs on Weight Loss and Plant-Based Eating

Many beginners wonder if a plant-based diet can aid in weight loss. Research shows that individuals following plant-based diets often consume fewer calories while still feeling full due to the high fiber content of fruits, vegetables, and whole grains. This means you can lose weight naturally by focusing on whole, unprocessed foods and being mindful of portion sizes.

Another frequently asked question concerns the sustainability of weight loss on a plant-based diet. To maintain weight loss, focus on developing healthy eating habits rather than strict dieting. Creating balanced meals that include plenty of vegetables, healthy fats, and whole grains can help you maintain your weight while enjoying the benefits of plant-based nutrition.

# How to Deal with Transition Difficulties

The transition to a plant-based diet can be challenging, but there are practical steps to ease the process. Start by incorporating more plant-based meals into your diet gradually. Try "Meatless Mondays" or replace one meal a day with a plant-based option. This incremental approach allows your palate to adjust while making the shift less overwhelming.

Additionally, plan your meals ahead of time to avoid the temptation of defaulting to non-plant-based options. Preparing a week's worth of meals or snacks can make it easier to stick to your new diet. Keep a variety of fruits, vegetables, grains, and legumes on hand to create quick, satisfying meals, and explore new recipes to keep things exciting.

# Concerns about Cost and Accessibility of Plant-Based Foods

One concern for many beginners is the perceived cost of plant-based foods. However, a plant-based diet can be budget-friendly when focusing on whole foods like beans, rice, and seasonal vegetables. Buying in bulk and shopping at local farmers' markets can significantly reduce costs. Prioritize whole foods over processed vegan products, which can be more expensive.

Accessibility can also be an issue, particularly in food deserts. To navigate this, consider joining community-supported agriculture (CSA) programs or seeking local co-ops that offer fresh produce. Many communities have initiatives to increase access to affordable fruits and vegetables, so research local options that can help you maintain a plant-based diet without breaking the bank.

# Strategies for Overcoming Boredom with Food Choices

Boredom can lead to a lack of enthusiasm for a plant-based diet. To keep your meals exciting, explore diverse cuisines that emphasize plant-based ingredients, such as Indian, Thai, or Mediterranean dishes. Experiment with herbs and spices to enhance flavor, and try new cooking techniques to discover different textures and tastes.

Additionally, make it a point to try a new fruit or vegetable each week. This not only keeps your meals varied but also introduces you to new flavors and nutrients. Creating themed meal nights, such as "Taco Tuesdays" with plant-based fillings or "Stir-Fry Fridays," can make your eating experience more engaging and enjoyable.

# Common Nutrient Concerns and How to Address Them

Many beginners worry about getting enough essential nutrients, such as protein, iron, calcium, and vitamin B12. To address protein concerns, include a variety of legumes, nuts, and whole grains in your meals. For iron, consume lentils, chickpeas, and fortified cereals, pairing them with vitamin C-rich foods like citrus fruits to enhance absorption.

Vitamin B12 is a common concern in plant-based diets since it's primarily found in animal products. To ensure adequate intake, consider fortified foods or a B12 supplement. For calcium, focus on dark leafy greens, almonds, and fortified plant milks. Educating yourself about nutrient sources can help you create balanced meals that meet your dietary needs.

# Tips for Maintaining Motivation and Consistency

Staying motivated can be challenging, but setting clear goals can help. Create short-term and long-term objectives, such as trying a certain number of new recipes each week or increasing your fruit and vegetable intake. Document your progress and celebrate small victories to keep your motivation high.

Joining a community or finding a buddy who shares your plant-based journey can also provide support. Participate in online forums or local groups focused on plant-based eating to share experiences, recipes, and tips. This connection can reinforce your commitment and provide inspiration to stay consistent with your dietary choices.

## The Importance of Self-Compassion in Dietary Changes

Practicing self-compassion is crucial during dietary changes. Understand that slip-ups are a normal part of the process, and be gentle with yourself when they occur. Instead of dwelling on mistakes, focus on the positive choices you've made and view setbacks as opportunities for growth and learning.

Cultivating self-compassion can also help you develop a healthier relationship with food. Rather than seeing food as a source of guilt or anxiety, recognize it as nourishment. Engage in positive self-talk and remind yourself of your reasons for choosing a plant-based diet, reinforcing your commitment to your health and well-being.

## How to Recover from Setbacks

Setbacks are a common part of transitioning to a plant-based diet, but how you respond is key. If you find yourself reverting to old habits, take a moment to reflect on what led to the setback. Analyze the situation, identify triggers, and consider how to approach similar scenarios differently in the future.

To recover effectively, return to your original goals and recommit to your plant-based journey. Reassess your meal plans and reintroduce variety to reinvigorate your diet. Remember, it's essential to view the journey as a process rather than a destination, allowing yourself the grace to learn and grow along the way.

## Engaging with Experts for Support and Advice

Engaging with nutrition experts can provide valuable insights and support as you navigate your plant-based journey. Consider consulting a registered dietitian specializing in plant-based nutrition who can help tailor a plan that meets your specific needs and goals. They can provide evidence-based advice on nutrient intake and meal planning.

Additionally, seeking out workshops, webinars, or cooking classes can enhance your understanding of plant-based eating. These resources can introduce you to new recipes, preparation techniques, and community support, making your transition smoother and more enjoyable. Engaging with experts can empower you with the knowledge and skills needed to succeed in your plant-based lifestyle.

## Recognizing the Long-Term Benefits of a Plant-Based Diet

Understanding the long-term benefits of a plant-based diet can help reinforce your commitment. Research indicates that plant-based diets are associated with lower risks of chronic diseases such as heart disease, diabetes, and certain cancers. Focusing on whole, nutrient-dense foods can improve your overall health and contribute to a longer, healthier life.

Moreover, a plant-based diet often leads to improved energy levels and better digestion due to higher fiber intake. As you transition, take note of the positive changes in your well-being, such as increased vitality and mood improvements. Recognizing these benefits can serve as motivation to stay committed to your plant-based lifestyle.

# Creating a Personal Action Plan for Ongoing Success

To ensure ongoing success, create a personal action plan that outlines your goals, strategies, and milestones. Start by setting realistic, achievable goals, such as increasing your vegetable intake or experimenting with a new recipe weekly. Write down your goals and refer to them regularly to keep your focus.

Incorporate strategies for meal planning, grocery shopping, and recipe exploration into your plan. Track your progress, celebrate achievements, and adjust your goals as needed. Having a structured plan can help you stay organized and motivated, making the transition to a plant-based diet smoother and more sustainable over time.

# CHAPTER 9:

## Conclusion and Next Steps

## Recap of the Benefits of Plant-Based Nutrition

Plant-based nutrition offers numerous health benefits, including reduced risk of chronic diseases, improved digestion, and enhanced energy levels. Consuming a variety of fruits, vegetables, whole grains, legumes, nuts, and seeds can provide essential nutrients while helping to lower cholesterol and blood pressure. This diet is also linked to better weight management, as it is often lower in calories and high in fiber, which promotes satiety.

In addition to physical health benefits, a plant-based diet can positively impact mental well-being. Studies have shown that individuals consuming more plant foods report lower levels of anxiety and depression. Moreover, this lifestyle can contribute to environmental sustainability by reducing carbon footprints and resource consumption associated with animal farming.

# Encouragement to Keep Learning and Experimenting

Adopting a plant-based diet is a journey of discovery that encourages you to learn and experiment with new foods and cooking methods. Start by exploring various cuisines that emphasize plant-based ingredients, such as Mediterranean or Asian dishes, which can introduce you to new flavors and textures. Don't be afraid to try unusual fruits, vegetables, or legumes, and embrace the creativity involved in preparing your meals.

As you progress, consider keeping a food journal to track what you enjoy and what works well for your body. This practice can help you refine your dietary choices and discover recipes that become favorites in your plant-based repertoire. Remember, the goal is not to achieve perfection but to enjoy the journey of exploring nutritious options.

# The Importance of Community Support and Resources

Connecting with a community that shares your plant-based interests can provide motivation and encouragement. Look for local meetups, online forums, or social media groups where you can share recipes, tips, and experiences with others. Engaging in discussions can also help you discover new resources, such as cookbooks or blogs that focus on plant-based cooking.

Consider joining cooking classes or workshops that focus on plant-based nutrition. These events not only enhance your skills in preparing plant-based meals but also allow you to build relationships with like-minded individuals. Community support can make the transition easier and more enjoyable, providing a sense of belonging as you adopt your new lifestyle.

## Setting Long-Term Health Goals

Establishing long-term health goals can help guide your journey toward a sustainable plant-based diet. Start by identifying specific areas you want to improve, such as increasing your intake of vegetables, reducing processed foods, or incorporating more whole grains. Setting measurable and realistic goals, like aiming to include at least one new vegetable in your meals each week, can make your progress tangible and achievable.

Regularly assess your goals to track your progress and make adjustments as needed. Consider celebrating milestones along the way, such as successfully completing a month of plant-based eating or mastering a challenging recipe. By focusing on long-term objectives, you can maintain motivation and see the positive impact on your health over time.

## Embracing Flexibility in Your Diet

A rigid approach to plant-based eating can lead to frustration or burnout, so it's essential to embrace flexibility in your diet. Allow yourself to enjoy occasional non-plant-based foods without guilt, understanding that balance is key to long-term sustainability. This mindset can reduce stress associated with dietary choices and encourage a more positive relationship with food.

Experimenting with different plant-based foods and recipes can also introduce variety into your diet. If a certain dish doesn't resonate with you, feel free to substitute ingredients or try a different cooking method. By remaining open to change, you can create a personalized plant-based lifestyle that suits your tastes and preferences while promoting health.

## Tips for Continued Growth and Improvement

To ensure your plant-based journey remains dynamic, continuously seek opportunities for growth and improvement. Stay curious by exploring new recipes, ingredients, and cooking techniques. Set aside time each week for meal prep, which can help you save time during busy days and encourage healthier eating habits.

Engage with nutritionists or plant-based coaches who can provide personalized guidance based on your health goals. Regularly attending workshops or classes can keep your culinary skills sharp and introduce you to innovative plant-based trends. Staying proactive in your learning can significantly enhance your overall experience and satisfaction with a plant-based lifestyle.

## How to Stay Informed About Plant-Based Trends

Keeping up with the latest plant-based trends is crucial for maintaining enthusiasm and creativity in your diet. Follow reputable food blogs, nutritionists, and chefs on social media platforms to receive inspiration and stay updated on new recipes, cooking techniques, and nutritional insights. Subscribe to newsletters or podcasts that focus on plant-based living to enhance your knowledge base.

Participating in local food events or plant-based festivals can also expose you to new products, innovations, and ideas in the plant-based community. Networking with other plant-based enthusiasts can lead to exciting discoveries and create opportunities to share resources. Staying informed will help you keep your diet fresh and enjoyable.

# Importance of Celebrating Your Journey

Recognizing and celebrating your progress in adopting a plant-based lifestyle is vital for maintaining motivation. Take time to reflect on your achievements, whether it's mastering a new recipe, sticking to your dietary goals, or feeling healthier overall. Celebrate these milestones with a special meal or by sharing your accomplishments with friends and family.

Additionally, consider creating a visual representation of your journey, such as a scrapbook or a digital photo album showcasing your meals and experiences. This can serve as a reminder of how far you've come and inspire you to continue on your path toward optimal health through plant-based nutrition.

# Engaging with Local Farmers and Markets

Connecting with local farmers and markets is an excellent way to enhance your plant-based diet while supporting your community. Visit farmers' markets to discover fresh, seasonal produce and unique plant-based products. Engaging with farmers allows you to learn more about how your food is grown, fostering a deeper connection to your meals and the environment.

Consider establishing a routine of shopping at local markets or joining a community-supported agriculture (CSA) program. These initiatives often provide weekly shares of fresh produce, encouraging you to try new foods and recipes. By incorporating locally sourced ingredients into your meals, you not only enjoy fresher produce but also contribute to sustainable food systems.

## The Role of Mindfulness in Nutrition

Practicing mindfulness in your eating habits can greatly enhance your plant-based journey. Start by slowing down during meals, savoring each bite, and paying attention to your body's hunger and fullness cues. This mindful approach can lead to greater satisfaction with your food choices and help you recognize when you're truly hungry versus eating out of habit.

Incorporating mindfulness can also extend to food preparation. As you cook, focus on the colors, textures, and aromas of your ingredients. This can create a more enjoyable cooking experience and foster a sense of appreciation for the nourishing foods you are preparing. By practicing mindfulness, you can cultivate a deeper connection to your food and your body.

## Preparing for Potential Dietary Challenges

As you transition to a plant-based diet, be prepared for potential challenges, such as social situations or cravings for non-plant-based foods. Plan ahead for events by researching menu options or bringing your own dishes to share. Communicating your dietary preferences with friends and family can also foster understanding and support, making it easier to navigate social gatherings.

Additionally, consider keeping healthy snacks on hand to help manage cravings or hunger pangs. Whole fruits, nuts, or homemade energy bars can provide quick, nutritious options that align with your plant-based goals. By anticipating challenges and preparing strategies to address them, you can enhance your confidence in maintaining a plant-based lifestyle.

## Encouraging Others to Explore Plant-Based Living

As you embrace plant-based nutrition, share your journey and experiences with others to inspire them to explore this lifestyle. Host a plant-based cooking class or a casual dinner party featuring delicious plant-based dishes that showcase the variety and flavor of this way of eating. Engaging with others can help demystify plant-based cooking and encourage them to try it themselves.

Moreover, share resources, such as books or documentaries, that have positively influenced your journey. Encouraging discussions about plant-based nutrition can spark interest and curiosity among friends and family. By sharing your enthusiasm and knowledge, you can contribute to a broader movement towards healthier eating habits.

## Resources for Further Reading and Exploration

To further enhance your understanding of plant-based nutrition, explore various resources available for learning. Numerous cookbooks and online platforms provide extensive recipes, meal plans, and nutritional guidance tailored for beginners. Websites and apps focused on plant-based eating can offer meal tracking tools, grocery lists, and cooking tutorials to simplify the transition.

Additionally, consider joining forums or online communities where you can connect with others pursuing a plant-based lifestyle. Engaging in discussions and sharing experiences can deepen your knowledge and help you stay motivated. Utilizing these resources will support your journey toward optimal health through plant-based nutrition.

# Common Concerns and Detailed FAQs

## Conclusion

Adopting a plant-based diet is a journey toward better health, sustainability, and ethical living. By understanding the fundamentals, building balanced meals, and addressing common concerns, beginners can confidently embark on this lifestyle. With continuous learning, community support, and a flexible mindset, anyone can thrive on a plant-based diet and enjoy the numerous benefits it brings to both personal health and the planet.

9 798301 005640